BEAUTY IS FOREVER

The Mature Woman's Guide to Beauty

I0450241

Joni Powling

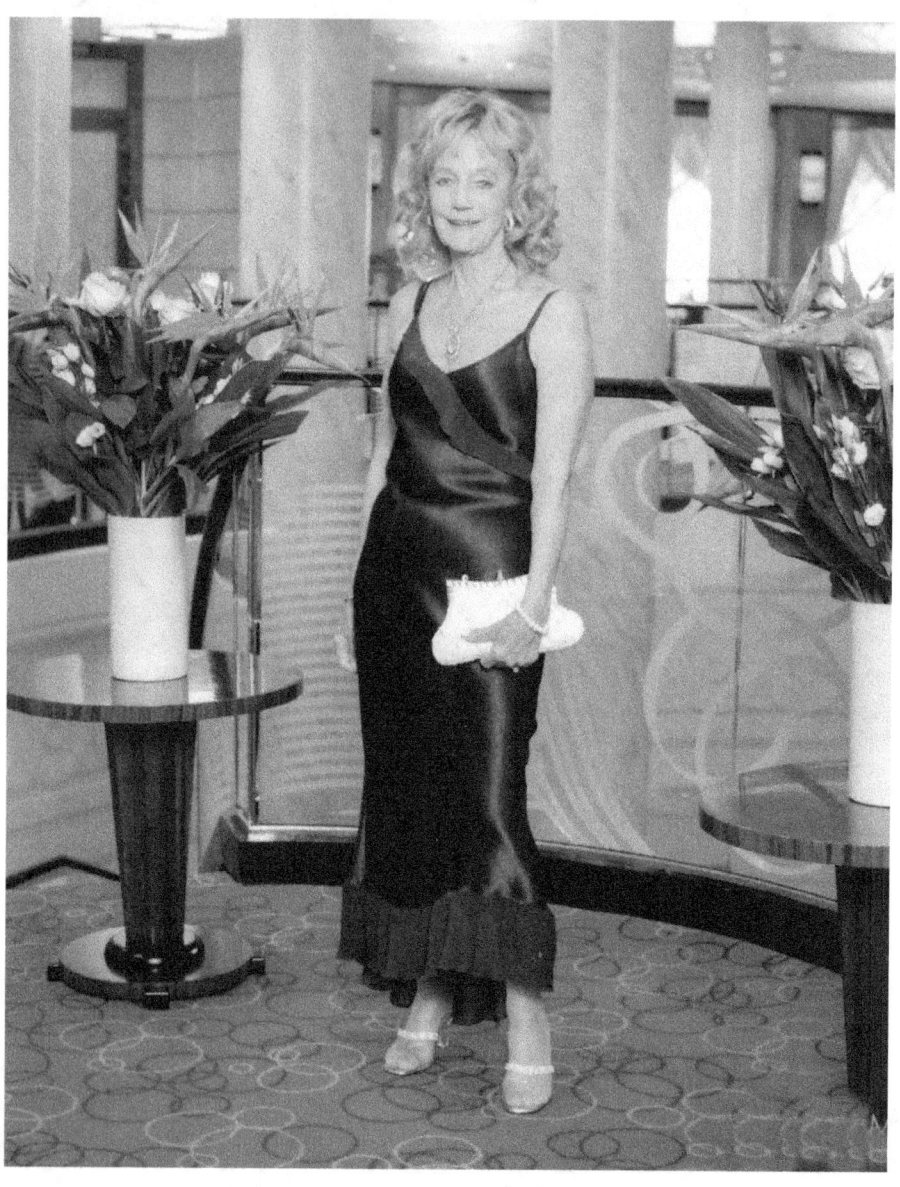

BEAUTY IS FOREVER

Joni Powling

First Print-on-Demand Edition April 2016

This book may not be reproduced in any form,
in
whole or in part, *without permission from the author.*

This book is dedicated to my son Peter whose support during the tough times has been my inspiration.

To my many American friends who, by means of long transatlantic calls, have confirmed their belief in me as a writer.

Last, but not least, many thanks to all the women who have read
Beauty Is Forever ... I hope you really enjoyed it and are looking forward to my next novel Dark Whispers from My Past, which will be available towards the end of the year.

Contents

Preface

Most women have a mid-life crisis and I was no different. Well, to say I was no different is stretching the truth a little, because, I don't think many of you would just up sticks and emigrate to another country; in my case America! Especially on your own with no contacts over there and, more importantly; no job to go to and precious little money in your pocket, but I had hopes and dreams – I had three diplomas packed in my case and the world was my oyster, so to speak, but fate has a way of turning our lives up-side down, just when we think we have got it right, and I soon found that America's streets were not paved with gold as we are often led to believe.

However, my fourteen years spent in

America certainly were not wasted, and, as I look back on that period of my life, I realize, more and more, how coincidence – chance meetings, etc., etc., can have a far reaching effect on our lives but, at the time, we simply do not realize it.

My landlord looked at me; his eyes betraying the pity he had for this English lady who was struggling to meet the rent every month.

But why couldn't I? Armed with a diploma in Reflexology, an international diploma in anatomy, physiology and body massage, etc., I thought I was in a good position to support myself but this was not the case. I had not done my homework before setting off on this great adventure, because if I had, I would have discovered that you cannot go to the United States with qualifications from another country as this would not be acceptable. You have to go back to school and get qualified in the State that you intend to practise in.

The outcome of this dilemma was solved when my landlord revealed that he was the owner of a large Beauty School in Hollywood and, according to him, I would find it far more lucrative to become qualified in the beauty business than anything else.

As he said proudly, 'Beauty is big bucks kid and don't ever forget it.'

Those few words changed my life forever as a whole new world opened up in front of me and finally ... *Beauty Is Forever* was born!

Introduction

My love of writing prompted me to write this book, together with a burning desire to help women to make the best of themselves no matter what their budget – we can't all be rich and famous! But, at the same time we can make the best of what we have.

The beauty business today is too complicated, too brash and too hard selling. The market is flooded with false claims about products that are extortionately priced and simply do not work! For two years now I have carried out extensive research and you will be shocked to find out how you have been misled by some of the most famous cosmetic houses, and how dangerous some of their products can be.

This is the reason I gave up my profession and decided to become a writer. I wanted to let people know the truth behind the hype, so that they would be in a better position to decide for themselves, what they should, or should not buy.

It is such a jungle of contradictory facts out there, that it is almost impossible for the average woman to find the time to plough through it all, much less understand some of the jargon! They are blinding us with science!

Now, I know how confusing it can be sometimes when we go to buy make-up. There is far too much choice today. All the cosmetic companies tout their products as being the best on the market. Well, of course they do! They want to sell their products so they can make as much money out of you as they possibly can –

that's business! But, it leaves you, the customer, bewildered as to what you should buy.

Recently I carried out a survey and asked a number of women if they were happy with the choice they had in make-up. Approximately 75 per cent said that they were overwhelmed by the huge range of cosmetics on display and, instead of being encouraged to buy, it put them off and they often walked out of the shop without making a purchase.

I am not now in the beauty business per say. I am now a writer who wants to give you, my readers, the best information I can on how to look good when we reach middle-age and beyond. I do not sell products so I have no financial interests in recommending any particular brand. If I do recommend anything, it is because either I use it myself, and therefore

I know whether or not it does what it claims, or I have done extensive research on that particular product. I also look at whether it is value for money and more importantly, if it is pure enough to go on your skin.

I do not have connections with any company that I mention in this book, what you are getting is my opinion and professional advice.

Chapter One

Sunscreen ... Should You Use It?

One thing in particular that really concerns me is the excessive amount of chemicals that can be found in some of the more popular brands of make-up. In fact, it is not only in make-up these chemicals can be found but in most beauty products, toiletries and many more.

Even if you have found something that you are led to believe is 100 per cent natural, it is quite possible that it is not. It may well have started out that way but, by the time the chemists have done with it – then it is a different story!

Most of what we read on the cosmetic label is misleading – in fact in some cases, it is a downright lie! The late Anita Roddick of Body Shop completely agreed with me on this point and I was very sad when I heard, later on, that Body Shop had sold out to L'Oreal/Nestle.

Just to give you an example, there is a popular brand of sunscreen that is currently on sale in the UK which contains over 46 chemicals. Just think for a moment, how many times in just one year alone you will apply this concoction of chemicals to your skin which will then be ingested into your body!

Why would anyone in their right mind, buy something that is full of chemicals, some of which could cause them a great deal of harm? Myself, I'll take my chances with the sun, at least I know what I am dealing with and can take the necessary precautions.

For years we have been advised to use a

sunscreen when we are going to be exposed to the sun and most people followed this advice faithfully. We were told that by following their guidelines it would reduce the rate of skin cancer.

But, let's look at the facts …

Since the invention of sunscreen several years ago, skin cancer rates are on the rise, both in this country and in the USA. In fact, according to the Office for National Statistics, in the UK the number of malignant melanoma exceeded 10,000 for the first time in 2010. If sunscreen is supposed to protect us against the UV rays then why is skin cancer steadily on the rise?

Would we not expect skin cancer rates to go down? Or is it more likely that it is the chemicals in commercially manufactured sunscreen which is causing this upsurge in cancer?

My research shows that during the past 10 years scientists studying cancer have come to the conclusion that some of the chemicals used in sun-screen may actually be increasing cancer rates. If they say that, you can be sure there's danger there!

In fact, during my stay in America I never used commercially produced sunscreen and I never developed skin cancer, yet a high percentage of my friends; the ones who were most meticulous about using sunscreen were, in fact, treated for skin cancer.

Doesn't it make you feel that there is something very wrong here? Even if you decide, for whatever reason, not to use sunscreen, you must make sure that you protect yourself with a sun hat and there are really some very glamorous ones out there, also protect your skin by wearing loose, light clothing with long sleeves to protect your arms. It is also essential to use a make-up that has an SPF of at least 15.

I have found a company called Green People that produces a sunscreen that comes up to my standards and I recommend it without hesitation. Their website address is greenpeople.co.uk and you can reach them by telephone on 01403 740350.

This brings me nicely to one point I would like to make and it is something I feel very strongly about. Whenever anyone tries to warn the public about the potential dangers of putting some of the substances contained in beauty products on the skin, there is an immediate outcry from certain quarters, denying that anything put on the skin can find its way into the body.

So … if this is the case, would these people care to explain to me how the contraceptive patch works when it is placed on the skin? Yet when it comes to beauty products we are told that the chemicals contained in the product cannot possibly be ingested into the skin!

I rest my case!

Chapter Two

You Can Have Perfect Skin at Any Age

It is amazing how many women go to bed without removing their make-up. No matter how tired you are, you must always clean your face before going to bed because this is the time the body rests and repairs itself.

Make sure you cleanse your face thoroughly and then apply a good toner. I would recommend Rose Water, which you can still buy from a few chemists; or you can find it on-line. It is quite inexpensive and does a good job of closing the pores of the skin. Why pay out pounds for a bottle of toner when you can buy Rose Water at a fraction of the cost and get the same results?

Moisturize, using one that is especially for your skin type. I personally never use anything on my skin that does not come up to my strict code of ethical products. Now, how you apply your moisturizer is very important and I never fail to be amazed at the way some women seem to just dab it on. You will get far more benefit if you first apply it to your décolletage then proceed in this manner; up the neck and then lastly onto your face, taking care to massage it in very lightly and always in an upward/circular movement until all the moisturizer has been absorbed. With the huge range of moisturizers on the market today, it's no wonder we look around us and feel totally confused with so much choice. Life was much simpler years ago, when you could go to the chemists or the make-up counter of a large department store and find just a handful of products to choose from. The way things are today, too much choice leaves us with no choice because it is so overwhelming.

During my career as a beautician I became increasingly aware that most moisturizers do not live up to their claims because the effect is only temporary! In a nutshell what happens is this:

Moisturizers add water to the outer layer of the skin (the epidermis). The effect of this is to plump up the skin as it begins to get more hydrated. Your skin feels softer and sometimes – after a period of use, you will notice a reduction in the fine lines on your face but this is only temporary. You need a product that may not be quite as dramatic as most moisturizers are in the beginning, but something that will gradually change the way your skin looks and feels over a period of time. That is what we are looking for – the long-term effect, not just a five-minute wonder!

I am not, of course, expecting you to be happy with a product that is going to take months to have any visible effect on your skin. I am talking about four to eight weeks, maybe even a little more if your skin really is very dehydrated.

When we pass our fiftieth birthday time is no longer on our side and we need to use products which are effective and simple.

Although I have given you advice on moisturizing your skin, I haven't used moisturizing creams for some time now. One of the reasons is that I don't like the feel of them on my face and it appeared that the more

I used them the more my skin seemed to dry out!

I have my own theory on that …

Now, I never buy any product just because of the manufacturers' claims. These companies are in the beauty business to make huge profits, so the wilder the claims, the more money that will find its way into their pockets. Sometimes we women are so gullible!

However, there is something on the market that I use and, I must confess, I am addicted to it. In fact to prove a point I will tell you the following story which is absolutely true.

Since my retirement from the beauty business I have lived in England. Recently, I received an e-mail from a couple of girl-friends of mine who live in the gorgeous little town of Naples on the Gulf Coast of Florida. They were about to take an extended trip to this country to visit family members and asked if I would consider meeting up with them and spend a couple of days at the beautiful Days Hotel in Bristol. Of course, I was delighted to be able to take a few days away from the pressures of writing and to catch up on all the gossip so I happily made my way to the hotel and met them in the lounge. After all the hugs and greetings were over, we retired to the bar for a glass or two of wine.

We had not been together for more than twenty minutes when they kept saying how good I looked! How much younger I looked! And that was before they had even finished one glass of wine! I didn't really take a lot of notice of what they were saying, especially as I had had a tiring journey – found I had left half my make-up in my bathroom at home and felt like a dog! My new shoes were killing me and my French designer trousers were definitely far too tight! Anyway we had a wonderful couple of days together and it was so sad to have to say goodbye to them once again.

When they finally arrived home they sent me an e-mail and here is an extract from it:

'We have just remembered another question we wanted to ask – your face looked absolutely fabulous when we saw you. Did you have some kind of face lift? If you did, tell us what kind you had. We know it was not the make-up because you hardly had any with you. Anyway, whatever you have done – keep it up – you looked wonderful. Whatever you did it took years off!'

For a few moments I could not, for the life of me, think what I had done to transform my looks to such an extent that they would rave about me like this. No-one had ever made such wonderful comments before (well at least since I have turned sixty). Certainly, I had not had any face-lift or any Botox treatments but then I remembered on that trip I had attracted the attention of two different guys who asked me for a date … I mean; they don't come that easy when you are past sixty …

Suddenly, it came to me. The only thing I had changed in my skincare routine since they last saw me was, instead of using a moisturizer as such, I had, in fact been using Almond Oil which, to be completely honest I absolutely love.

As I have said previously, it is very important to me that whatever I put on my skin must be the purest that I can find and price comes into it too. I work hard for my money and don't want to waste it on something that could potentially have harmful effects on my health or something that didn't do anything for me at all …

I have to say that I have changed since using it – my skin looks younger and plumper and it has got to do with the Almond Oil and my own special water regime' which is fabulous for beautiful skin.

At this point you are probably wondering,

if the regime' with the water was the secret of beautiful skin, then why am I also using Almond Oil! Why would I need it? That is a very good question.

Having lived in a hot climate for such a long time, my skin got a certain amount of sun damage and, I must admit that I have never used sunscreen in my whole life but I did get those horrible brown patches appearing on my face which are so difficult to cover up no matter what you use. Clear skin is beautiful skin; patchy, discoloured skin is not! I have to say that the Almond Oil is gradually, very slowly, getting rid of these patches and they are certainly less noticeable. By the way, it is said to be excellent for stretch marks and recent scars on the body but I haven't tried it in this aspect as yet.. Another thing in its favour … a little goes a long way.

If you use a little before putting on your make-up, be sure to apply it at least five minutes beforehand, because it takes that time to be absorbed into the skin and you do not want to apply make-up onto a skin that has surface oil on it.

There are two types of Almond Oil – Pure and Sweet Almond Oil – but the one I personally use is the Sweet Almond Oil which is very reasonably priced at around £3.95 per 100ml. I have listed below some of the benefits you can expect from using Almond Oil, but first let me warn you that it is a little heavy – so use very sparingly.

Here are a few more of the benefits of this lovely little oil:

1. It will give your complexion a lovely glow.
2. It delays the ageing process.
3. Dark circles around the eyes appear lighter.
4. Almond Oil also helps to relieve dry skin and it is excellent for nourishing your hair and your nails.

The only downside is that Almond Oil can turn rancid, so it is very important that you store it in a cool, dark place and once opened it must be stored in a refrigerator.

How often you use it is a matter of choice. I know of women who apply it just a couple of times a week who are quite happy with the results, while, on the other hand I have a few friends who use it nightly. Whatever you do, remember the advice I have already given you. Always cleanse your face before going to bed!

At this point there is a little story that I would like to share with you and I think that you will find it very interesting. Plus it will give you details of the water regime' which I have mentioned and that is virtually free! What could be better?

During my time in the United States I met many women; most of them were extremely wealthy and could afford to have any treatment they desired to enhance their looks, regardless of the cost. They all looked very glamorous with their designer clothes and immaculate hairstyles and, of course, their make-up was perfectly applied but only two women, a mother and daughter, stood out from the crowd, so to speak. They were not particularly wealthy; the mother was just an ordinary beautician until she decided to launch her own company selling natural skincare products. She also trained her daughter to help her in the business.

Within two years they became extremely successful and this was in a town where it was not the easiest place to start up a little beauty business. Competition was fierce and ruthless … but they had one thing in their favour that was priceless! When you met them, all you could do was to marvel at their skin. It was absolutely glowing, plump and moist without a blemish on it and, the most interesting fact of all was that the mother's skin was just as good as her seventeen year old daughter. The mother had no wrinkles, even though we were living in a very hot climate, which as everyone knows, can be so very damaging to the skin.

I wondered whether or not she may have had surgery but then discounted the thought. Even after having a face-lift you may not have any wrinkles but your skin doesn't plump up and look dewy and fresh like a teenager. I just could not figure it out. In this case, their success was due to the fact that they were living proof they had cracked the secret of beautiful skin.

When I got to know them better and we became friends, I asked the mother one day while we were having lunch, if she would kindly tell me the secret of her lovely skin. How was it that she had the skin of a teenager? In all my experience I had never seen anyone whose skin looked so fabulous. Immediately, I made up my mind, I wanted to look like her! I wanted to buy whatever she used! I didn't care what it cost!

Imagine my shock when she told me that her beautiful skin was not due to any expensive skin care products, or any secret recipe handed down from her grandmother – it was simply due to the fact that she kept it well hydrated with plenty of water. I looked at her and shook my head in disbelief. I didn't quite understand what she was talking about. When I want to cleanse my face I use soap and water not cleansing lotions, so I thought I was hydrating my skin and I told her so. She smiled, almost as if she felt sorry for me because I just didn't get it. Then she explained her routine…

Apparently, every morning without fail she would douse her face and neck with plain lukewarm water for five minutes. No more, no less! She would carry out this routine twice a day and had done so for many years. She had also instilled in her daughter the necessity of keeping the skin well hydrated and the results were amazing.

The face is what draws people to you and it is essential to keep it looking as good as you possibly can. As we age we become more dehydrated and water is our best friend. So many women today never put any water on their face – they are so indoctrinated by TV adverts that they are led to believe they need a cleanser to remove make-up.

Soap and water has been frowned on for many years by the cosmetic companies. We have been told that soap is bad for the skin. We were told soap is drying to the skin but what they don't tell you is that many, many of the products they advertise contain exactly the same chemicals as can be found in soap, except that soap has far less!

In fact soap has been a tried and tested way to cleanse the skin and it has been around for years and years … but there is very little profit to be made on a bar of soap. After all you wouldn't be prepared to pay a few pounds for a bar of soap would you?

So the word was spread around that soap was bad for the skin; it was very drying but a facial cleanser is kinder to the skin and doesn't dry it out. The cosmetic houses then put this, allegedly far superior facial cleanser on the market, and were able to charge you a lot of money and so it boosted their profit margin and that is all they care about! Of course, not all companies have this attitude and I have found some extremely ethical in their dealings with the public. But not very many!

There is no moisturizer/treatment on this planet that can have such a dramatic effect on your face as this simple water routine, regardless of what the big cosmetic companies may say. But, please remember this; you have to do your part to see the results. Apart from the water dousing there is another crucial element to help you retain great skin and a youthful look and that is to drink plenty of plain, filtered water. You should have at least eight 8-oz glasses a day and please cut down on the amount of juice drinks, high-calorie sodas and alcohol that you drink, as this will screw up your whole system.

As we get older, our need for water becomes more acute, because dehydration actually speeds up the ageing process. But, by drinking water you are keeping the blood volume high which enables it to reach all the little capillaries in your body. This, in turn, distributes nutrients and oxygen which keeps the cells youthful.

FOR GREAT LOOKING SKIN MAKE THIS A RITUAL YOU NEED TO CARRY OUT FOR THE REST OF YOUR LIFE – AND THE BEST PART IS THAT SO FAR YOU HAVE PUT VERY FEW CHEMICALS ON YOUR SKIN OR IN YOUR BODY! AND IT HASN'T COST A FORTUNE.

Another tip is to try to avoid drinking too much coffee as this is very, very dehydrating and so is not good for your skin, or for that matter your health.

I know how much you love to sit around chatting to your friends and drinking coffee and I am no exception but, if you must have your coffee, please take my advice and go for decaffeinated – that goes for tea as well. Also beware of the very popular energy drinks. Some of them contain as much caffeine as coffee – so you see your energy drink might not be as good for you as you are led to believe. What is the point of following my water regime to hydrate your skin if, at the same time, you are pouring drinks down your throat that are causing dehydration? You will only be going around in circles.

Your best bet is to stick to decaffeinated drinks and plain, filtered water. Your skin will begin to look good and the water is actually flushing the toxins out of your body at the same time. Now, you don't have to stick rigidly to decaffeinated tea or coffee – I know how difficult this can be – I have been there, done that! Treat yourself sometimes to your regular coffee or tea but don't make it a habit; just a couple of times a week.

You will see a vast difference in the way your skin looks and you will feel pretty good too!

Chapter Three

Exfoliating Is a Must ... But Beware of Eye Creams

As I have said previously, as we get older it is essential to keep the skin well hydrated. The flexibility of the skin depends entirely on its moisture and oil content and as we age there is an overall slow-down (as with the rest of our body) in our skin's ability to repair itself. It has less ability to regenerate new cells, so dead cells build up on the surface, giving it a dull, grey appearance which is not very flattering. Once these have been removed the skin immediately appears to be healthier and has more radiance. You can achieve this look by exfoliating the skin.

It always surprises me to find that so many women neglect this most basic and important part of skin care, even if you only do it once or twice a month you will see the difference. Not only does exfoliating the skin make it appear brighter and smoother it also removes impurities such as pimples etc.

REMEMBER: This is a gentle procedure and does not take away a whole layer of skin like some of the more popular but harsher procedures. It is quite simple to do this at home and all you need is to look in your kitchen cupboard to find the ingredients. You will also find it so much cheaper to formulate your own mixture than buying it commercially; plus it is so easy even a child could do it.

Here is my own recipe' which I have used

for several years:

Mix together 1/8th cup of oatmeal (organic if available), 2 tbsp milk, 1 tsp baking powder and a teaspoon of olive oil. Apply to a clean, dry face using half-circular motions with your hands making sure that you cover your neck and decollate' area as well. When you have covered all these areas, fill your wash-basin with tepid water and douse your face, etc., until you have completely removed all traces of the mixture ... pat dry then stand back and look at yourself in the mirror and see how much better and brighter your skin looks.

Before I leave the subject of skin care, there is just one more point that I would like to make perfectly clear to you, my dear readers, and that is not to become confused with the different procedures that claim to give you the perfect skin. Exfoliating the skin is a far gentler approach to perfect looking skin than say chemical peels. These are quite dramatic procedures which, in most cases use products which contain AHAs (alpha hydroxy acids) and BHAs (beta hydroxy acids) which dissolve the top layer of the skin.

Yes, you will look great afterwards, I don't dispute that but did you know that when you remove the outer layer of the skin, you also remove its protective barrier. This allows anything that comes into contact with the skin to penetrate into the deeper layers. You also remove the natural pigmentation which protects us against the rays of the sun and so, if you take away this protection, then the ultraviolet rays can cause considerable skin damage. Maybe even cancer!

Could this possibly be another answer to why skin cancer is on the rise? I personally have seen older women in the United States who have had so many treatments, over a period of time; their skin is like thin, transparent paper! It is not a pretty sight, so my advice to you is this …

Respect your skin and it will respect you.

You can look good without all these expensive procedures, plus you will be healthier without all the chemicals in your body. Of course, it is not possible to totally eliminate all chemicals because they are everywhere. In the food we eat, in the products we use in the home, also in toiletries, make-up and beauty creams and potions. However, we can reduce the amount we ingest into our bodies by eating sensibly and following my guidelines on beauty.

Now, there is one question that I am often being asked by women and that is whether they should use those eye creams that profess to eliminate fine lines and dark circles around the eyes.

This is something that I am in two minds about. Firstly, I have never used an eye cream as such. The skin around the eye area is so very delicate that you have to be very, very careful what you put on it. This can best be illustrated by the following situation that happened last summer …

My friend Jennie called to see me one day, she was worried because the skin around her eyes had become very puffy and she felt her eyelids were beginning to droop. As soon as she walked in the door she started … Jennie's like that!

'Why is it that your eyes are still alright?' she said, staring crossly into my face. 'After all you are years older than me – so why can't I have eyes that look like yours?' She paused for a moment to catch her breath then said sadly, 'I will have to have plastic surgery on my eyes now and I am only in my forties!'

I gave a deep sigh as I studied her face closely. She was right! Her eyes looked awful, so puffy and the lids were actually drooping, but I had seen such a situation a few times before when I was in the States and I just had to ask her one question to clarify what I believed to be the cause.

'Have you been using any cream around your eyes?' I asked.

She nodded miserably. 'But it was a cream

that was specifically for the eye area,' she protested.

'Well, I am sure that's your problem. What I want you to do is leave the cream alone – give your eyes time to recover but, if they feel uncomfortable, just put a couple of cold, used tea-bags on them and then see how you are in a couple of weeks.'

Jennie turned on me angrily.

'What are you talking about? I told you I have been using a cream that was advertised as solving the problem of puffy eyes, now you are telling me not to use it! I just don't understand.'

Jennie really doesn't have much patience!

'Just give yourself two weeks without creams around your eyes. Try the tea bags but make sure that you have steeped them in water first and squeezed out the excess, then come back and see me, I replied, as I guided her gently towards a chair so that she could relax while I talked to her.

'Jennie, don't believe everything you see advertised on the television or anywhere else for that matter,' I said. 'It's all about money. In fact one of the largest cosmetic companies made a profit of 1,653 billion Euros in one year alone – that is a lot of money by anybody's standards. This same company, along with several others, was ordered by the Therapeutic Goods Administration in Australia to stop advertising a wrinkle cream because it really did not do the job! Just think how much of their hard earned money women have wasted putting this product on their skin and getting nothing back. It's the same situation you have found yourself in now, except of course it has made your eyes worse!'

Two weeks later she arrived at my door with a huge smile on her face and, I must say she looked marvellous. Her eyes were looking fantastic, the puffiness had gone and with it the drooping of the eyelids. *And, best of all she didn't need surgery!*

Before Jennie left she turned to me and asked what I used around my eyes. I had to tell her the truth – I don't put any cream around my eyes that professes to take away lines and puffiness because for me they don't work. Maybe for some people they do – but for me they don't. The skin around the eyes is so very delicate that, more than any other part of the face, you need to be very cautious about what you use in that area and the minute you see some adverse reaction throw it away!

Now, when you reach our age group there is no reason to be obsessed with a few lines on the face – you will only end up by being very miserable, chasing the impossible.

Of course, you could have a face-lift and you would probably be very pleased with the result. But a face-lift only lasts between eight to ten years, then you need another and then another … and so it goes on until you end up looking worse than when you first started!

If you are very wealthy and are happy to go through these procedures despite the risks involved, then that's fine! I wish you well, but my purpose in writing this book was solely to help the thousands upon thousands of women out there who don't have a lot of money to spend on themselves. I know of women in both this country and the United States, who have never had a facial or any other beauty treatment in their life – but it doesn't mean that they don't care how they look – they just don't know how to help themselves and couldn't afford the expertise to help them along the way … until *Beauty Is Forever* appeared on the bookshelves.

Chapter Four

Make-Up Hints and Tips for the Over Fifties

Now that you have, hopefully, started to take good care of your skin we can move on to the question of make-up.

There is one thing in your make-up bag (or should be) that will take years off your looks, yet it only takes two minutes to apply and that is Yves Saint Laurent Touche'Eclat. I know it's a little pricey but it will last for ages.

By the time you reach the age of forty, your eyes will begin to show signs of age. It's natural and happens to all of us. The skin around the eyes starts to get thinner and very often dark circles start to appear.

Now, I am not saying that this happens to everyone, because it doesn't but I am preparing you for the possibility of having to deal with such a situation. Nothing is more ageing than dark circles around your eyes … you need to use a good concealer/brightener and yet I would go as far as to say that only a small percentage of women in our age group are using a concealer.

Even if you don't have dark circles, you will find that as you get older the skin around the eye area becomes darker, or, in some cases redder than the rest of the face and that is ageing!

If I were given the choice of only one item of make-up that I could use, it would be a concealer that is light enough to use around the eyes and as I have said Yves Saint Laurent is definitely one of the best on the market. It makes me look well rested and it certainly takes years off my looks. Nothing is as powerful at reducing the signs of ageing, or as quick to apply.

Look in your mirror now and study your eyes.

Do you see what I am talking about?

You may have a perfectly made-up face, but if you have not used a concealer around your eyes, then you have wasted your time? Well! Maybe not totally – but you could look better – you could look at least ten years younger!

Now, eye make-up is something older women are very uncertain about and I have been asked several times whether or not it is the 'done thing' to wear mascara or eye shadow when you reach say sixty and beyond. This is my own personal view gained from years of experience making up older women.

Eye make-up has become big business over the past few years and yet I can remember years ago, when all you could find on the make-up counters was block mascara in probably black, brown and maybe a midnight blue. If you were lucky there would be a few pots of eye-shadow in even fewer colours. Now, these days the choice is overwhelming, to say the least and the amount of different mascaras all claiming to do something magical for your lashes is phenomenal. Most of them do not live up to their promise but, of course, if you were to wear false eyelashes, then the mascara would create the same effect that we see advertised on the television however, mascara alone cannot produce those long, lush lashes unless, of course, you have been gifted with really good strong lashes, and then you are very lucky!

But what do women of our age group do about such issues? We don't want to look ridiculous but, at the same time we would all love to have long, thick lashes. So I decided to test the water, so to speak, on your behalf and I experimented with different mascaras, then I tried individual false eyelashes that you apply yourself – but they kept falling off! Finally I decided to have them done by a lash technician. Well, they certainly did not fall off! They will stay on until your own lash, to which each individual fake lash is applied, falls out … the only trouble was that I did not like myself with a full set of fake lashes and it is taking months to get rid of them.

I could go back and have them removed professionally, but then I thought of the strong chemicals that would have to be applied in order to remove them and I didn't really fancy that. So I have come to the conclusion that you can get away with a full set of fake lashes when you are young but not when you are older, although I must admit I now put just a few fake ones at the outer corner of my eyes and that looks fantastic because it opens up the whole area …

But all this doesn't mean that our eyes have to be as nature intended. I am a fanatic about my mascara and I certainly would not go out without it. It certainly enhances my eyes but most women in our age group, unless they are a celebrity, as a rule do not wear mascara every day.

Maybe they will put a little on when they go out for a social evening but that is about as far as they will go; especially when they get sixty and beyond. But why not? What is wrong in making the best of yourself? What is the difference between thinking it is okay to wear lipstick at our age but mascara is a big NO!

I believe this is all down to the fact when we were growing up there was very little choice in make-up and certainly mascara seemed to carry some sort of taboo. Apparently it was accepted if you were a film-star or an actress etc., but 'nice girls' did not wear mascara. The trick is to apply a thin layer of a non-waterproof mascara to your lashes, then when that has completely dried, apply another thin coat to the outer top lashes. Of course this will not apply if you have decided to have a few false ones placed in the corner as I have suggested, but make sure that you do apply mascara carefully to the remaining lashes. This will help to 'open up' your eyes thus giving a more youthful appearance, but it will be subtle and, therefore, suitable for any age.

You are probably wondering at this point why I advise non-waterproof mascara and the reason is this. I have found that if you use waterproof mascara it tends to give a much harsher appearance to the face. When you are young you can get away with it – but when you are older you can't! Also to remove the waterproof mascara you need to buy a remover especially formulated to do the job and, in some cases, this can cause a severe reaction while, on the other hand, ordinary mascara can be removed quite easily.

Before I leave the subject of eye make-up, there is one product worth mentioning and that is L'Oreal Paris Lash Renewal Serum. If you use it constantly for a few weeks you will find that your lashes look longer and stronger – it also makes your lashes look thicker.

There is just one thing I want to warn you about … some people, in fact, quite a few, have had an allergic reaction to this product so if you experience any stinging or irritation around the eye area after using it please stop straight away. Bathe your eyes in lukewarm water and realize that this product is not for you. However, if you are able to use it then you will find a great improvement in the length and thickness of your lashes. How do I know that this stuff really works? Because it has been tested by several of my friends in America and they rave about it. I tried it myself recently, purely for research purposes but, I was allergic to it and when my eyes started stinging I knew it was not for me.

To frame your eyes you must take care of your eyebrows. Now, I know that it is a problem when your eyebrows are getting sparse and the colour seems to have faded but, there is a solution to these problems. As far as I am concerned, the best way to achieve fabulous eyebrows is to have them tattooed, but, of course, you must find a technician who is well qualified in eyebrow tattooing. More and more beauty parlors are offering this service but be sure and check that the technician who will be carrying out the procedure has some experience under their belt.

Remembe: when it is done there is no going back.

It is pretty expensive and prices can range from £300 to over £1,000, so it's not a procedure to be taken lightly.

If you don't fancy having your eyebrows tattooed then do as I do! Brush your eyebrows with a powder which matches, as closely as possible, to your own colour. A slightly darker shade will give more definition to the brows.

Follow the arch of the eyebrow with an eyebrow brush then gently seal them with a little wax to keep the hairs in place. You will have glamorous eyebrows all day long with this procedure and it is the cheapest way to go.

Foundation

It is notoriously difficult to find a foundation that actually makes you look wonderful although there are a million different ones out there that claim to do just that. Unfortunately, many of us get swayed into buying a product purely because of the way it is marketed. Well, of course, that is the sole purpose – to encourage us to buy! Glamorous women stare at us from our television sets, telling us how, by using this particular product, we can look as flawless and beautiful as they are … and I must admit they do look absolutely stunning.

We go into a store to buy some make-up and we see the same beautiful women staring at us from bill-boards…it is hard to resist isn't it? But you will never look like that in reality, no matter what your age, because the models have been professionally made-up; then air-brushed and they are young; few of them are over the age of thirty. So what works for them cannot, and will not work for you in the same way.

I have one golden rule for our age group and that is to avoid heavy foundation. Too many women seem to think that the thicker the foundation the better they will look. This is not true! It will clog your skin and emphasis lines in your face … In other words it is ageing when you reach a certain age.

Another point to remember is to apply your foundation in a good light and make sure that you take the foundation onto the neck and décolletage so that it all blends together. During the day get a hand-held mirror and stand in front of a window where there is a good light. This is particularly important when you are buying at a store because the fluorescent lighting, which is so common today, gives a totally fake image of how you would look in natural daylight. This is why, before you buy any new make-up, you should check it out in daylight; most stores will gladly give you a small mirror to take outside, then you will get a true picture of how you really look.

Personally, the only foundation I would ever use is Id Bare Minerals because it is so light that you feel you are not wearing any make-up at all and it is pure. It has the ability to transform mature skin by covering up all the imperfections. I have had many compliments about my skin but truthfully, it is not that brilliant, it is the Id Bare Minerals that makes it look perfect, yet, at the same time it gives the impression that I have hardly any make-up on at all. This is one product that you should really try, but let me give you a word of advice, read the instructions on how to apply it correctly, don't treat it as you would an ordinary face powder … The secret is in the application.

Now, before I leave the subject of make-up I would just like to talk a little about lip gloss. This is a definitely a NO! for older women.

For example, by using lip gloss you are drawing attention to the mouth and that is something you do not want to do when you are in your sixties, seventies or even older. We are trying to conceal those tell-tale little lines around the mouth, not emphasize them! What I suggest is that you use a lip liner pencil in a colour slightly lighter than the lipstick you are using, and then when you have outlined your lips use a nice, light moisturizing lipstick and blend it into your liner.

One of the very best things you can do for your lips is to use a good lip balm and the best time to use it is the last thing at night, just as you are about to retire.

There is a very good organic lip balm on the market that I use which really helps to hydrate your lips and it also helps with those little lines around the mouth. It is produced by a company called Miessence based in Australia where their Jaffa Lip Balm was guaranteed through the Australian Certified Organic party. Which, of course, means that their products do not contain any synthetic chemicals or pesticides, nor do they test their products on animals?

Back in 2008 the Natural Skin Care Product Review rated a lip balm manufactured by a well-known company as being highly toxic and they are not the only ones to be guilty of this. Remember, whatever you put on your body finds its way into the body!

Now, if you are really worried about the little lines that appear around the mouth, and then by all means go to a qualified practitioner who specializes in lip enhancement if you wish … But it is very expensive unless, of course, you have a husband or boy-friend that would be willing to foot the bill!

Then there is the problem that it is extremely difficult to find a really competent person. When I talk about being competent, I mean not only someone who is qualified, but someone who also has an artistic streak in them – someone who can mould your lips to suit your face and your age. Too many practitioners out there today are competent in giving the necessary injections but they haven't got a clue beyond that.

My firm belief is that only qualified persons in the beauty business should be allowed to do lip enhancement and fillers. After all, we have to study long and hard to become beauticians and we are trained to look at a face as an artist would look at his painting. We can recognize the simple little touches that will enhance someone's appearance. Not all practitioners in lip enhancement can do that!

You only have to look at some of the celebrities we see on the television these days to see what I am talking about.

Chapter Five

Face-Lifts and Fillers

Many women are opting for a face-lift these days and I agree that in the first few months, or even up to a year you will look absolutely fabulous, providing, of course that you have found yourself a very experienced surgeon to do the job.

But your face doesn't stop ageing once you have had this procedure. Sadly, a lot of women seem to think that once they have had a face-lift they never have to worry about looking old again … This is not true! Eventually little lines will start appearing within a year or two after the procedure, according to your own personal rate of ageing and, between eight to ten years you will find yourself needing another face-lift and so it goes on and on, until one day you wake up and find that you look worse than you did in the beginning.

The trouble is that these same women do not seem to think that it's a big deal; but the truth of the matter is, that it is a big deal! In fact, it is major surgery and carries as many risks as open heart surgery and no-one wants to go through that, do they?

Years ago it was a much simpler operation because the surgeon only cut into the skin and then pulled it tight to get a reasonable effect but nowadays, it is far more complicated – surgeons are now cutting much deeper through the skin and also through the nerves and arteries. Sometimes, it can happen that as you heal, skin tissue can shrink and this necessitates another operation, which in itself can cause more problems.

Instead of taking all these risks and facing such an invasive procedure my advice to you is to go for one of the facial toning and firming devices. There are several on the market and I have tried one or two but the one that I really like is the Tua Tre'ndface. This will, by electrical stimulation, actually tighten up the underlying muscles of the face and neck.

Consequently, after a week or two you will find that your face and neck appears toned and more youthful. Lines are gradually fading and you can actually feel your skin becoming firmer. In fact, a look in your mirror will tell you that it really works, but apparently if you stop using it your face will start to show signs of ageing.

Before you rush out to buy a Tua Tre'ndface I would like to give you a little advice. You may find it difficult to get used to at first. I know I did! But, it does not take very long to get the hang of it – just be a little patient. Also, there are contraindications which, of course, mean that some people who have certain health problems should not use it. To save you the trouble of perhaps ordering one and then finding that it is unsuitable for you, I have decided to list the contra-indications below:

- Pathological facial conditions
- Pacemakers
- Metal pins and plates
- Neurological disorders including epilepsy or multiple sclerosis
- Weak psycho-physical conditions

- Broken or bruised skin
- Large protruding atypical moles

If you are not sure always check with your doctor.

Now, I would like to talk a little more about fillers. Years ago animal based collagen injections were all the rage but then it was found that some people were allergic to these products; which were derived from cows. Then they tried filling in wrinkles and contouring the face with fat taken from your buttocks but that was not really successful …

The filler I would recommend (should you wish to go down this road) is Restylane which has practically no risk of an allergic reaction. Restylane is made of hyaluronic acid, which occurs naturally in the human body. This filler works best for lip augmentation and fine wrinkles. The hyaluronic acid in Restylane attracts water molecules to the area thus filling it in. Even better is the fact that it will last between six months to a year. The price of Restylane per syringe is between £400 and £670 but if you can afford it, then I would say that it is money well spent.

There is one other filler that I would recommend and that is Radiesse. It is filler which is best suited for the deeper wrinkles on your face, especially the nasolabial folds which run down from the nose to the mouth. It is made up of a calcium material and can last from between two to three years but, the downside is that it costs almost double that of Restylane. However, the choice is yours and if you are unhappy with lines on your face and want a quick fix — there is no better way.

Now, before I go on any further I want to bring the question of silicone being used on the face and whether or not it is safe.

I have done extensive research into the dangers of silicone upon the body — in fact I would class myself as somewhat as an expert in this field as I have had first hand experience of it being put into my body and I want to tell you emphatically it is a dangerous substance that should not be allowed anywhere near the human body.

It has caused untold misery to millions of women, especially the ones who have had breast implants. Too many people in the medical profession and the cosmetic industry will tell you that it is an inert substance ... that's fine when it's not going into your body and you are making a lot of money from it. But try telling that to the millions of women who have suffered debilitating illnesses, even death through breast implants!

Now, when we get into our late fifties or so, we start to panic about it. Suddenly it's upon us … and we start to feel old.

I know that some of you out there will be reading this and saying 'I don't feel old and I am fifty-eight!'

Well, then I am pleased for you and hope this feeling will continue throughout your mature years, but I know that you are in the minority. Most of the women I have come into contact with over the past few years, dread and agonize over the fact that they feel they are old!

This really is a critical time in a woman's

life…she is desperately searching for some magical potion that will restore her youth, or, maybe some talented surgeon who could sweep away the years with his scalpel. Failing that she will look to the anti-ageing creams to solve her problem and the sad thing is that they really don't work as well as they say and they will cost you a fortune!

There is a way to get a good anti-ageing treatment for your face and neck which is cheap and does not contain dangerous chemicals and that is the Sweet Almond Oil.

This lovely little oil contains Vitamins B1, B6, and A plus a few others and it works by refining the structure of the skin; it also stimulates cell renewal.

It works well for both dry and sensitive skin, in fact it is good for all skin types.

D0 NOT USE IT IF YOU HAVE A NUT ALLERGY.

Chapter Six

My Secret to Eternal Youth

Dealing with the problem of ageing means more than just worrying about a few wrinkles and here is my advice…

Stop counting the birthdays – after all age is just a number. You can look fifty at thirty-five and, equally, you can look thirty-five when you are in your fifties so why fret and worry about your age? The more you worry about it … the quicker you will age.

When I reached sixty, I decided that I did not want anyone to remind me of my age. So family and friends were told that the quickest way to upset me was to send a birthday card with my age on it. To me there is nothing worse – I hated those cards.

Who wants to be reminded that they are coming to the close of their life? Why celebrate that you are another year older? Don't get me wrong! I love to get cards from my family or anyone else who cares to send one … but, please not any with reference to my age. I hated it when friends or family reminded me that I should apply for a bus pass.

I couldn't imagine anything worse. It might save me a little money but it would ruin my self-esteem. All these things make you feel old!

Now, there is nothing wrong in wanting these things but it is not for me. For years I have held the belief that looking young for your age is just as much about your mind and how you perceive getting older, as it is about what you wear and your outlook on life. Remember! You are as old as you feel …

IT'S A PACKAGE DEAL!

I am always being taken for being a lot younger than I really am, and the reason for this is because I follow the guidelines in this book.

The mind and body connection plays a big part in staying youthful. For example if your brain is absorbing messages that you are getting older, it then influences your body with this in mind.

I know some people will not agree with this point of view and they will insist that it is all to do with our genes. Yes, of course, our genes do have a lot to do with how long we live etc., but I believe, and I am living proof that my theory works, that our brain gives out signals to our body based on the information it receives. For example, if we are constantly thinking 'old', then your brain processes this thought, and passes it to your body which starts to age.

We have all been in that situation when we don't feel too good and promptly take ourselves off the see the doctor. It's all gloom and doom isn't it? The doctor writes out a prescription and you totter off to the chemist to get this magical cure.

On your way there you run into an old friend who looks you up and down and says, 'How are you? Say! You look really good!' Immediately you receive a rush of the feel good endorphins and, as you continue your trip to the chemist, you realize that you don't feel sick anymore! In actual fact you feel great!

The answer is that your friend changed your thought pattern and your body has responded accordingly.

It works all the time!

Only last week I went into my local Post Office feeling reasonably healthy but, because I met a friend in there who said I didn't look very well, that I looked very pale (she should try being a writer!), I came out feeling decidedly poorly – she had spoiled my day … Because she had changed my thought pattern.

A few days ago I received a telephone call from a lady who is ninety years old. I know her quite well and have, from time to time, travelled to her home in Somerset to give her a complete make-over.

Yes, even at ninety, apparently we still

worry about our appearance! Anyway, during the telephone call she asked me if I could please come over and see her as soon as of possible and try to do something with her face – she was feeling a little depressed with herself.

Now, this lady was the sort of person, who thought a little lipstick was enough, until one day she asked me what I did to make myself look so good. When I explained my regime' to her and then followed it up with a complete make-over, she looked like a new woman and no-one would think she was ninety!

She was so pleased with the result that she took me out to dinner that evening and, as we sat in the restaurant enjoying a glass of wine, she told me that, knowing she looked as good as is possible for her age, made her feel much more confident and happy.

The moral of this story is that how we look affects our entire body, either in a positive or negative manner depending on how we see ourselves. When we look in a mirror and see ourselves looking good it makes us feel happy, thus creating the rush of endorphins, a chemical which is created in the brain. This chemical really gives us a boost which creates confidence and a feeling that all is right with our world.

So you see how important it is in our later years to take care of ourselves, then we can have the 'good feel' factor all the time.

No matter what your age remember … Beauty Is Forever!

Chapter Seven

The Secret Behind Thicker, Healthier Hair

I don't believe that it's all down to ageing when we see so many older women with thinning, dull, lacklustre hair. I am also aware of the fact that we can't hope to have hair that is as gorgeous as we had in our twenties and thirties, but there are a few things we can do to change this.

I went through a period in my life, actually it was when I was in America, that I got so fed up with my hair I bought a wig and wore it for several months. My own hair had become dry and unmanageable and seemed to be thinning at the crown. I was devastated because I had always been very fortunate to have a really good strong head of hair and I had many compliments on it – now all I wanted to do was hide it under a wig!

The trouble was that I really didn't stop to think how very uncomfortable a wig might be in the sub-tropics and, it was not until I actually started wearing one and the temperature soared to over one hundred degrees, that I realized a wig may be great in England in our cold, rainy weather – but in a hot country – forget it! So I decided to solve the problem of my hair by doing some extensive research.

It didn't seem right to me that, with all the modern shampoos, conditioners and all the other aids for glamorous, thick, healthy hair, so many women were suffering with hair problems such as dryness, shedding and itchy scalps. It just didn't make any sense to me, especially when you realize that more and more women are suffering from hair loss and other related problems today, than at any other time in our history.

I remember my grandmother who, at the age of 86 years, had lovely long, silver hair. My mother was exactly the same; she had thick, healthy hair right up until the day she died…so what was their secret? It is quite simple really – they did not use hairsprays, conditioners, hair dyes or any modern products. When they rinsed their hair, they would add a few drops of either vinegar or lemon to the last rinse to balance the ph levels of the scalp; which is the first step towards healthy hair. Lemon juice is best for fair hair and vinegar is for dark hair.

Obviously, it is important to get your hair in good condition but that is not easy these days. We are battling with fluoride in our water every time we wash our hair.

Fluoride is an enzyme poison and the body can only eliminate about half of it. It is very damaging to the thyroid gland and studies show clearly that it causes many health problems – including hair loss! The best way to avert these problems is to have a water filter fitted to your tap which will remove about 99 per cent of the fluoride.

Then there are the chemicals in hair products, shampoos, conditioners, hair-dye and hair sprays etc. etc…

It's almost like a mine-field out there! And, I must admit that I was shocked at some of the things I uncovered during my research.

For example: sodium laurel sulphate is just one of the numerous chemicals found in many popular shampoos, hair conditioners, toothpaste and body wash. It is a strong, harsh detergent commonly used as an engine degreaser. My research showed that using products containing this chemical can cause problems. For example it can cause severe irritation to the eyes. It can also cause skin problems, especially if you have sensitive skin and, even worse…it can cause hair loss!

Another interesting thing I discovered was a chemical called isopropyl – sometimes marketed under the name of alcohol. This is a poisonous solvent found in some hair colour rinses. It was also extremely interesting to discover that it is known to cause dry skin and HAIR! Yet it is to be found in some hair conditioners!

Rather strange, don't you think? What is

going on out there?

Are we, the consumers caught on some sort of merry-go-round?

We buy products that are touted to solve a certain problem, yet, in some cases the very product we bought is, in fact, actually compounding it!

I believe there is some very clever, if not right down devious, marketing going on and my point in bringing this to your notice is simple. These are just two of the many chemicals found in products commonly used and they create havoc with the health of your hair. So, is it any wonder that, after several years of putting these chemicals on our hair, it's going to start to get thin and loose its lustre?

Your hair might look good now – but what's going to happen when you have used these chemicals constantly on your hair for several years?

Some of the most popular brands of hair dyes and shampoos that we buy in our local high street store contains these chemicals, so check before you buy!

It is, of course, possible that the condition of your hair is caused through a health problem and, in that case, you should be seeking medical advice.

Personally, I have found that taking silica (which you can get from your local health store or from your local Boots) works wonders for your hair and nails but you still need to be very selective about the products you buy. Another product to consider is Kelp tablets which supply the body with all the nutrients required for thick, healthy hair. After all, as we get older we do seem to get a little short of the necessary nutrients our body needs for optimal performance – so give it a little help along the way. In the meantime, avoid any product like the plague if it contains any of the chemicals that I have mentioned above or indeed, any of the ones listed in my final chapter.

This is the first step on the road to recovery for your hair and, although it's not going to be a 'quick fix' it will, in time, pay huge dividends.

There are shampoos which do not contain these chemicals – although I must admit that even some of the 'all natural' ones may contain some of them. The one I would recommend, and which I use myself, is intensive repair shampoo (for coloured/treated hair) produced by Green People. It contains plant extracts and essential oils which will infuse your hair with vitality and shine.

There are, of course, other good products which do not contain dangerous chemicals but just make sure you take the time to check the labels. I know it's a pain and we shouldn't have to waste our valuable time reading them, and the least we should expect from manufacturers of such products is that they are safe to put on our hair, or for that matter, what we put on our skin. Unfortunately, it's not quite working that way and they are not being honest with us. In fact, I would go as far as to say that they are definitely putting profits before people!

We all know how important it is to condition your hair after shampooing but there is no need to waste your money on commercially produced ones and you can also save yourself the trouble of looking at labels if you use what I recommend.

When you get to our age it is important that, as well as price, we find something which is going to be kind to our hair, so my advice to you is use mayonnaise as a conditioner but don't go for the reduced fat one? The mayonnaise original is perfect and it is so simple. Just apply a small amount to your hair before washing it then massage the mayonnaise in with your fingers, making sure you pay particular attention to the ends. Cover with a shower cap, wait for ten minutes before rinsing and then wash your hair thoroughly with warm water. It really is a remarkable conditioner and this is due to its high content of egg yolk, oil and vinegar … all these ingredients are so good for the hair and can't do us any harm. Which reminds me of a popular saying … If you can't eat it; don't put it on your body.

Another tip on home-made conditioners is to use an egg. Just beat it for a moment or two then add about a tablespoon of tepid water (make sure it's not hot water or it will solidify the egg) and apply to damp hair, massaging into the scalp.

Leave on just for a minute or two before rinsing with warm water. If you leave the egg on your hair too long it will be difficult to remove. I use both these conditioners depending how I want my hair to look. For example when I use the egg, I find that it makes my hair appear to be much thicker and it has a lot more body than when I use the mayonnaise. Whereas, using mayonnaise seems to make my hair softer and shiny. It's all about personal choice.

When you condition with either the mayonnaise or the egg, you are putting fatty acids and vitamins into your hair, making it stronger and healthier as against putting chemicals on your hair; which will cause it to become weak and dry. But, if you don't fancy coating your hair with mayonnaise or egg then I suggest, as an alternative, you try the olive oil method.

Now, I am a great fan of olive oil, it is especially good for people with dry hair. Just massage a small amount of the warm oil into your scalp and hair, cover with a plastic shower cap, or, failing that put a warm towel around your head and leave it for as long as possible before shampooing. Keep in mind that when you are going to shampoo – make sure that you put the shampoo onto your hair before you add the warm water; otherwise it will be very difficult to create lather.

I often wonder why some women will go to the trouble of buying expensive hair oils, when olive oil does the trick just as well – in some cases even better and, what's more it works out much cheaper. However, if you don't want the bother of preparing your own conditioner then once again I would recommend the Intensive Repair Conditioner by the Green People.

Dandruff

If you suffer from dandruff your hair will always look dull and dry but, don't worry, there is a simple remedy and you can probably find it in your food cupboard. What is this magic ingredient? Well, it is our old friend vinegar.

You can use either apple cider vinegar or distilled white vinegar, they are both equally effective and you will find that your scalp feels cleaner and fresher even after just one application.

Mix equal quantities of your chosen vinegar and warm water and apply to the scalp. One of the best ways of doing this is to use a spray bottle but, if you don't have a spray bottle handy then just put it in a jug and pour it over your hair.

Squeeze out the excess then wrap a towel around your hair and leave for a few minutes, then shampoo and rinse well.

Within the space of two or three applications you should find your scalp clean and free from dandruff…plus you have saved yourself some money!

If you suffer from greasy hair, use Apple Cider Vinegar as follows:

After shampooing and rinsing dilute 2 tablespoons of apple cider vinegar in a large cup of warm water and pour it over your hair – you will certainly see a difference but please do not do this more than twice a week, especially if you have a sensitive scalp.

Are you worried about hair loss?

I have been researching a natural product for hair loss and I would certainly recommend this to anyone who is seriously concerned about the amount of hair they are loosing.

The product is called Provillus and is marketed in a pill form. The prominent herbs to be found in Provillus are saw palmetto and nettle which help to block (DHT) dihydrotestosterone which is responsible for slowing down hair growth. The herbs in Provillus work by feeding the follicles in the scalp, therefore, encouraging new hair to grow. If you do decide to try this product, then you will be pleased to see that there is a money back guarantee – so what have you got to loose?

Another remedy for thinning or loss of hair was given to me years ago when I was in America. During the time I was there I spent a lot of time with the Seminole Indian tribe in the Everglades of Florida and I got to know them very well. We talked of many things but the one thing that struck me most of all was their total commitment to living off the land; both for their food and also their medicine and toiletries.

One day while sitting in a chickee (which is an open-sided palm thatched hut). I asked one of the women how they managed to have such beautiful, shiny hair and it was so thick and strong. She just smiled at me, then, taking me by the hand she led me to a green, prickly plant growing a few yards away from the hut. Bending down she broke a stem and then broke it in half again and a clear, thick liquid started to ooze from it. She rubbed the liquid between her hands before putting it on her hair; pointing to me indicating that I should do the same.

This is the secret of the Indians fabulous shiny hair and the plant was the aloe vera.

On my return to England I researched the

plant and found that it contained over 20 amino acids also vitamins A.B1, B2, B6, B12, C and E. When it is applied to the scalp it restores the ph balance and also adds nutrients to the hair roots and follicles. What a wonderful little plant this is!

Before I leave the subject of hair, I would like to share with you one of my pet hates. A few years ago there was this feverish trend which sent most women under the age of sixty to her hairdresser to have her hair bleached and straightened until there was not as much as a kink in it. *Women everywhere looked the same – it was almost as if they had been cloned! Whatever happened to individuality? Why are women today so desperate to look like their favorite celebrity?*

The last time I went to a hairdresser, I was made to feel like a freak because I have wavy hair and I want to keep it that way. No amount of persuasion was going to change my mind. When the assistant was working on me, I realized that this young girl did not have a clue how to style. She was only competent at straightening hair, that's all she had ever done, so after my appointment I came out of that salon looking like a demented poodle. The sad fact is that today we have very little choice unless of course we are getting married or we go to a very high priced salon, then and only then will they come up with a decent style!

Our choices are long, straight hair – which does not suit older women or, maybe I should rephrase that and say it only suits a small minority of older women, or, as is more fashionable, the short bob worn by Victoria

Beckham.

At the time of writing the long, straight hair is gradually being replaced by long, wavy hair. But, if you are on the wrong side of sixty – you have no choice – it's the old 'granny' style for you. It may be different if you have the money to go to a top London salon but if you have to rely on your local hairdresser, that's what you will get! Unless, of course, you are lucky enough to have a hairdresser who actually listens to you.

Looking fantastic as you get older is not just a question of getting your hair and make-up right, or for that matter, having plastic surgery or botox. As I have said previously – 'it's a package job', and by that I mean that you need to take a serious look at yourself then answer the following questions:

1. Take a look at the clothes that you wear. Are they dark and dowdy? A bit frumpy!

2. On the other hand, are you trying too hard to say young by copying trends that are designed for someone years younger than you?

3. Have you changed your hairstyle in the past five years?

4. If you wear spectacles, are they modern and trendy? Or are you still sticking with the ones you had ten years ago?

5. When you are out – do you walk tall?

6. Are you applying the mind and body connection?

These are just a few of the points that you need to address if you want to look great at any age

...

First of all let us look at the clothes the average older woman wears. It is my opinion that 50 per cent of women in this country do not make the best of themselves (remember that I am talking about the older generation now, not the younger ones).

When I came back to England, after the time I spent in America, I was shocked to see that most women wore trousers – it was almost like a uniform but, at the same time not a very flattering one and the reason for this is that so many women these days are overweight. Yes, there are times and places where trousers would be perfectly acceptable, for example if you were going on a hike through the countryside, or when you are going to the supermarket ... but, please make an effort when you are going out for the evening. Nothing looks more elegant than a skirt either long or short, it doesn't matter. Just take a break from wearing trousers constantly.

Chapter Eight

Fashion Tips for the Over Sixties

The first rule to remember is to avoid wearing 'granny' clothes. By this I mean the ones that you hide behind, because they give you the feeling of having a comfort blanket wrapped around you. You need to step out of your own private box and invest in some new clothes. Don't be afraid that they may seem, to you, a bit daring, a little too young for you, or the colour is too vivid … but, believe me, if you stop making excuses and act upon my advice it will take years off you.

Too many women tend to wear mainly black or beige – sensible clothes they may be – but also very boring. It is also very important to find your own personal colour code and this can be done quite easily by going on-line and go into Google, then type in colour coding and you will get up a site that will instantly give you all the information you need to know what colours really suit you.

Another little tip is stop wearing anything that has a rounded neck as it does not do anything for women of our age. Whether you are buying a dress or a top it makes no difference, the style you need to look for is the v-shape neckline. It flatters older women because it elongates the neckline and seems to make you look taller and slim.

Underwear

Almost 80 per cent of women are still wearing the type of underwear that they wore in their twenties and thirties and that is a big mistake. As we age our bodies change and it needs a bit of support in certain areas. We all get that annoying tummy problem: What happened to that lovely taunt, attractive tummy we used to have in our teens and twenties?

It has gone the same way as the boobs, the bat-wings etc., and it is up to us to do something about it. Of course, there is surgery, but I would not recommend it. First of all it is so costly and secondly it can be dangerous.

What you need to do is invest in Lycra Control Wear or sometimes called Magic Underwear. It will transform the way you look when you are dressed … even if you are overweight it will still do its job and your body will be transformed. This in turn will boost your self-confidence and you will feel and look like a million dollars.

Hairstyles

Don't be afraid to colour your hair … you are never too old to look glamorous. Obviously you couldn't wear some of the extreme hair colours that we see today, but you can go with a colour that is similar to that which you had before it started to go grey and you won't go far wrong. If you would like a complete change of colour then opt for a shade a little lighter than your original hair colour – that will also work very well and you will be surprised at how much better, a simple thing like changing your hair colour, will make you feel about yourself.

When it comes to styling my advice is that there are just two things to avoid when you reach sixty and over. The first is that having a tight perm is a big NO! It is so ageing and it's no good trying to make yourself look younger by following my advice on make-up and clothing if you are going to spoil it all with your hair looking like a cork-screw. If you really must have a perm, then go for a very soft one that looks natural.

Secondly, do not wear your hair longer than level with your chin. Or, if you have long hair and don't want to have it cut – try wearing it up. If you abide by these rules you can have any hair style you fancy and you will look great.

Do you need to wear glasses?

Now let us take a look at spectacles. Unfortunately it's when we reach the age of fifty or beyond that we start to notice how small the print is getting when we try to read the newspaper or our favourite magazine. To solve the problem we buy a pair of reading glasses and then spend the rest of our lives looking for them!

I drove my family crazy by constantly wandering around the house complaining that I couldn't find my glasses, so, in the end I decided that the best thing I could do was to go for contact lenses. After all if they were in my eyes I couldn't loose them – or so I thought! Happily I made my way to the opticians and not only did I come away with a pair of contact lenses, I came away with a pair that were tinted blue which greatly enhanced the green of my own eyes and the effect was stunning.

Unfortunately, they didn't solve my problem and I soon discovered that it is quite easy to loose a contact lens during the process of putting them in or when you take them out. Once that happens it is almost impossible to find them, then it's back to the opticians again. Finally, I made a decision to have Lasik surgery and that was the best thing I have ever done. It was virtually painless, I could see perfectly within a few hours and I didn't have the problem of loosing anything so I was happy.

Regarding price, you will find that it starts at around £395 per eye and remember that I said 'starts' at £395 approximately. The price will be set according to the eye exam results that you will have to have before the optician can begin his work. The price can escalate to £1,000 or so according to the condition of your eyes, so be sure to clarify the cost after you have had your eye exam and before any treatment begins or you may be in for a shock.

Walk tall

One of the biggest give-away of age is the way we walk. Approximately 70 per cent of women over 65 walk badly. Now, I am not targeting the people who have a health problem because, unfortunately, they cannot help it but there are thousands of women out there who have no excuse and it's time to straighten up and walk tall.

The best way to achieve this is to set up a routine. When you are ready to go out, stop for a moment before you open the door and consciously straighten your spine, tuck your tummy in and stretch your head up from your shoulders ... then you are ready to face the world. After a few weeks of practising this routine you will find it comes naturally and people will suddenly begin to notice you.

The mind and body connection

Have you noticed that overweight women are always going on about their weight? They tell anyone who will listen that they hardly eat anything and yet they still put on weight. I have a friend who is in that category and I know for a fact that she eats far less than I do and yet I still retain the same weight as I was in my teens, which is exactly 112 lbs. My friend is constantly on a diet of some sort or another but it makes no difference – she still remains overweight. I have never dieted in my life and I can eat anything I like without having to worry about putting on weight … so why is this and what is the answer?

My theory is that it is the mind and body connection.

In other words whatever we constantly think about in our brain will manifest itself in the body. For example, when I was growing up I constantly worried about being too thin, all my friends had puppy fat and I was like a greyhound. I would look in a mirror and agonize over my too thin body.

My friend looks in a mirror and sees an overweight lady and that picture is immediately picked up by her brain which then responds to her thought process which is an overweight woman. If she could only persuade herself to think differently, and instead of worrying about her weight just keep a picture in her mind as being thin, then, I believe she will start to loose weight. There is jut one point I would like to stress here and now. If you have a health problem that is causing you to put on excess weight, you need to take your doctor's advice.

Now, I realize that a lot of my readers will think I am crazy but I know you can control your body with your mind because your body responds to the way you feel, think and act. I have put this into practice in other areas of my life and it really does work …

It takes time and commitment but the results are worth a king's ransom.

Remember, the simplest things are usually the most effective!

Chapter Nine

The Toxic Chemicals in Skin Care Products

It is never too late to start taking care of your body and no matter what age you are … you can start NOW!

Beauty begins with a healthy body.

In this chapter I am going to talk a little about the amount of chemicals still being used in make-up etc; even though there is increasing evidence to show that these chemicals can create havoc with our health. While millions and millions are spent on research for cancer we are getting nowhere regarding the cause and I firmly believe that the chemicals in the products we use every day are a contributory factor to this and other serious health problems. For example, consider the following.

Sodium lauryl sulfate

This is commonly used as an engine degreaser, as a garage floor cleanser and it is also found in toothpaste, body cleansers, shampoos and bubble bath. It is a dangerous substance which is found in over 90 per cent of personal products.

In fact it was while I was in America that I found that some toothpastes carried a warning, which they have to do by law, because they contained sodium laurel sulphate and it stated:

'Warning. Keep out of the reach of children under 6 years of age. In case of accidental ingestion seek professional assistance or contact a poison control centre.'

They don't put out warnings like this for fun!

As sodium lauryl sulfate is easily absorbed by the body, it can do irreparable damage to the heart, liver and brain so think about this when you have your next relaxing bubble bath! Or even when you next shampoo your hair! Because, unless you have been very selective in your choice of shampoo, you have a 75 per cent chance that the one you are using has sodium lauryl sulfate in it.

Acetaldehyde

This is a known and suspected carcinogen (a cancer causing substance) yet it is put in some of the products we use. It is easily absorbed through the skin and is very toxic. Acetaldehyde has been found to cause kidney damage and in some people it can cause a serious allergic reaction. Acetaldehyde is very destructive of the mucous membrane and the upper respiratory tract, eyes and skin.

With so many people suffering from sinus problems – it makes me wonder!

Ammonium lauryl sulfate

This again is a potent chemical that is used in products to produce foam. It is also known to irritate the eyes, skin and mouth of some people. It is in many shampoos and bubble bath products, in fact anything that creates foam will, most probably contain this chemical.

Aluminium salts (aluminium chlorohydrate)

Used in antiperspirants and deodorants, they work by creating a coating over the sweat glands. Possibly linked to breast cancer; which as everyone knows is on the rise in both this country and the USA where people use the most deodorants.

Aluminium has also been linked to Alzheimer's disease, so go easy on deodorants and opt for ones that are far less toxic to the body.

DEA (diethanolamnine), MEA (monoethanolamine) and TEA (triethanolamine)

Used in some cosmetics, face and body creams, these are harsh solvents and detergents and tests have shown they can cause an allergic reaction in some people. Long term use can cause kidney and liver problems.

Isopropyl alcohol

This is used as a solvent in many of the products you can buy over the counter. It can cause a nasty skin irritation and it actually strips the skin of its protective acid mantle.

Parabens (methyl, propyl, butyl, etc.)

Widely used by the cosmetic houses to extend the shelf life of their products, it is estimated that approximately 13,000 cosmetic and skin care products contain parables.

They are extremely toxic and can disrupt the hormonal processes in the body and can cause problems with the endocrine system. A recent UK scientific study shows there was a specific link between parables and breast cancer.

When you look at the labels on any beauty product that you buy you will find that almost all of them contain this deadly substance.

In fact, according to the US Environmental Protection Agency, these chemicals displayed estrogenic activity in several tests and it is well known in the medical profession that estrogen stimulates breast cancer. They also found that anything absorbed through the skin may be as high as ten times the concentration of an oral dose. I am convinced that the majority of cancers are caused through the amount of chemicals we are exposed to day after day and we need to do something about it.

Propylene glycol

Used as a carrier in fragrance oils and also as a moisturizer in cosmetics. Propylene glycol can cause kidney and liver abnormalities.

Formaldehyde

This is a known carcinogen and can cause an allergic reaction in some people. In studies it has been linked to contact dermatitis, headaches and chronic fatigue.

It is interesting to note that chronic fatigue is a condition that has doctors baffled, and yet the amount of people complaining of symptoms relating to this condition is rising each year – but still we don't know what causes it! Maybe they should concentrate on the serious effects formaldehyde can have on the unsuspecting public!

The problem is that we are constantly being assured that the amount of these chemicals in any one product are of a minimal quantity and cannot do us any harm.

(*Where have I heard that phrase before?*)

But no-one seems to be able to explain that if we are using the 'safe' limits each and every day, year in and year out, then we must obviously be getting an 'overdose' and that, I believe, is when the body starts breaking down. We also use more than just one product per day that contains these poisons. So, people who use these commercially produced products are ingesting a huge amount of toxins into their body day, after day, after day ...

At this point you are probably wondering, if these toxins create such havoc with our bodies – why the manufacturers still are using them. The answer is simple and it is what has caused to most of our problems in the world today ... GREED!

You see the products I have mentioned are relatively cheap and easily available so it means more profit in the pockets of the manufacturers and that is all they care about. Well, not all of them but a large majority and my research shows that it is some of the well known and trusted companies who seem to be the worst culprits.

Remember, the only safe chemicals are

the ones you are not in contact with.

Another point to remember is that anything you put on your skin will find its way into the bloodstream and become integrated into the body tissue.

It is impossible for me to list all the dangerous chemicals found in products we use and I have only documented a few – but I hope it will make you more aware of the dangers you face every day in your pursuit of beauty and that you will, in future, take the time to check labels. Better still; buy your products from ethical companies. You will find the companies I recommend in this section of *Beauty Is Forever*. Nothing is more precious than your health and the health of your loved ones.

It is up to you to check what is in your make-up, toiletries etc., and, if you're not happy –

don't buy it!

Chapter Ten

Safe Sunscreen for Everyone

First of all, I want to emphasize that some of the top cosmetic houses are the worst offenders when it comes to adding chemicals to their products. They are charging the earth for their make-up and toiletries – they seduce you into buying with glossy advertising and, very often, false claims and your well-being comes pretty close to the bottom of the list I'm afraid.

Green People's organic sunscreen range is a non pore clogging natural sun cream and is the one that I recommend for those of my readers who do not want the bother of making their own.

Many others contain mineral oils and silicones that form an impervious synthetic barrier on the skin…which is akin to wrapping your skin in cling film!

I don't think you would like to do that. Would you? The other plus in buying Green People's sunscreen is based on the fact that, because of its purity, it is suitable for people with sensitive skin.

They also have an organic sunscreen combining SPF 15 with a tan accelerator which contains an extract from the carob tree; this speeds up tanning naturally by 25 per cent and reduces tan fading by almost 50 per cent … This is a product well worth trying.

You can buy it on line at organic@greenpeople.co.uk – or you can contact them by telephone on 0140374035.

Another company that I recommend is Welder and you will find their products in most Health Stores also Boots. Their telephone number is 0115 944 8222 or you can reach them on their web site sales@weleda.co.uk.

Make-up

First, I want to talk a little more about moisturizers. If you really like the idea of slathering cream on your face then make sure you check the ingredients list shown on the product. If, and most certainly it will, contain any of the chemicals I have warned you about, don't buy it!

Some of the well-known companies actually contain a substance that is known to cause dry skin. You would be far better off using simple olive oil or the sweet almond oil that I recommended earlier. Olive oil has been the choice of many famous women, past and present, who have used it to protect and nourish their skin.

Another point in its favour is that it is so pure and free from harmful chemicals.

Now, Bare Minerals make-up is without a doubt the choice for a lot of older women (me included) because it looks so natural that people will comment on your beautiful skin, but the truth is it's the make-up that creates the illusion. Bare Minerals is free from chemicals and toxins and, if you have never tried them, now is the time.

You can contact them on 0800 6523362 or by e-mail at

customer services@bareminerals.co.uk.

Of course, there are many more companies out there who are excellent and who use organic and ethically sourced products but, the ones I have listed are the companies I personally use and I can vouch for them. Just be aware, if you are shopping around for cosmetics or toiletries, that, although something may state on the label it is organic, this doesn't necessarily mean that the product is totally free of chemicals.

As I have already mentioned, there is growing concern that certain chemicals found in many brands of deodorants, on sale in this country, have been linked to breast cancer – I think it's best to err on the side of caution and be sure to check before you buy. Or, failing that, go with one of the companies that I recommend.

Making your own sun-screen

It really is quite simple to make your own sun-screen and this tip was given to me by a good friend when I was in the United States. Unfortunately, I did not meet her until I had been living there for two years and, had happily sunbathed with very little protection whatsoever. Obviously, my skin did get a little damaged but this recipe protected me from further damage.

Buy plain zinc oxide ointment and just mix it with your preferred skin lotion and apply whenever necessary – but be aware that zinc oxide is a powder and you must take care not to inhale it. You will not only be saving money by making your own sunscreen but are drastically reducing the amount of chemicals you ingest… It takes a long time for chemicals to build up in your body – you may be feeling fine now. But, stop for a moment and consider how you might feel in 5 to 10 years time?

If you do not want to go to the trouble of making your own sun-screen then follow my guidelines and you will be doing the best you can for your skin and also for your health.

One of the most important things to remember is that beauty is not just about applying make-up, having botox or a face-lift … or even having a wonderful wardrobe of expensive clothes – beauty is the whole and not just a part of the body and that means taking care of the inside as well as the outside. Looking young for your age is not solely about having a wrinkle free face – as I have said before in this book … It's a package deal!

How do I know all this? Because I am

constantly being taken for someone twenty years younger, no-one believes me when I give them my age and that is without ever having a face-lift or botox etc. For several years now I have faithfully followed all the guidelines that I have given in this book.

It's never too late to start ... You will be amazed at the results.

Author Biography

A broken marriage and a sudden desire to start a new life in America changed Joanne's life forever. From a rather drab existence in rural England she found herself in the sub-tropics … in a town called Hollywood.

With little money and no contacts she began to forge out a future for herself in this tropical paradise.

Two years later she was a qualified beautician with wealthy clients and life was good. Life was exciting…But paradise does not last forever and an unrelenting desire to return to her roots took control of her and, after spending a total of ten years in paradise, she 'came home' with the words of her clients ringing in her ears ...

'Please put all your beauty secrets in a book so we will be able to follow your advice, even if you are over 3,000 miles away.

So ... Beauty Is Forever was born ...

www.ingramcontent.com/pod-product-compliance
Lightning Source LLC
Chambersburg PA
CBHW062008280526
45787CB00005B/2024